I0842686

OSTEOPOROSIS REVERSAL
DIET COOKBOOK

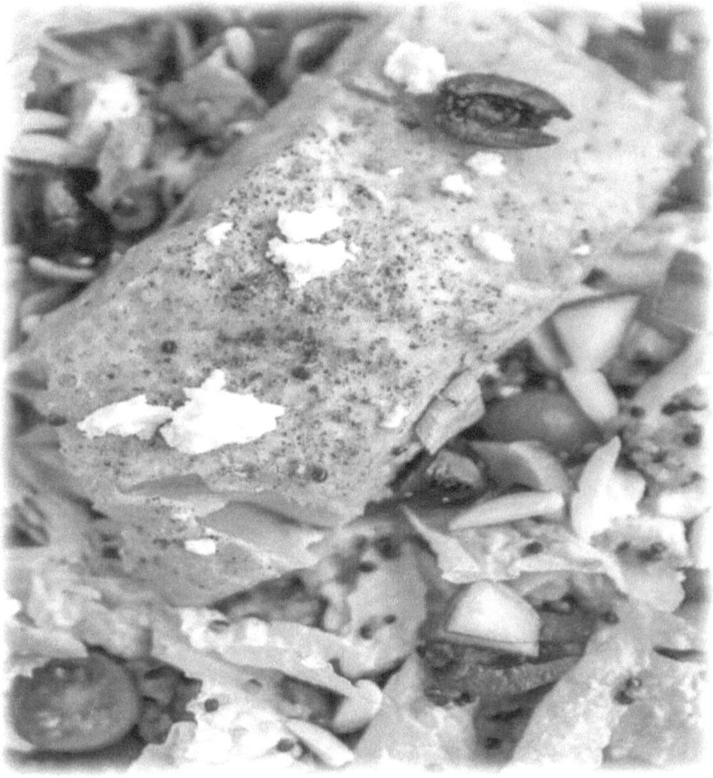

Easy To Prepare Calcium-Rich Recipes for

Healthy Strong Bones

LAKEISHA OWENS

Copyright @ 2024 by **LAKEISHA OWENS**

All rights reserved. No part of this book may be reproducedin any form or by any electronic or mechanical means,including information storehouse and reclamation systems,without authorization in writing from the publisher, exceptby a critic, who may quote brief passages in a review. Thisbook is a work of non-fiction.

Published in 2024

TABLE OF CONTENT

More..................

More....................

INTRODUCTION

Osteoporosis, a skeletal disorder characterized by weakened bones that are more prone to fracture, affects millions of individuals worldwide, significantly impacting their quality of life. Recognizing the pivotal role of nutrition in bone health, the "Osteoporosis Diet Cookbook" emerges as an essential guide for those looking to fortify their bones through dietary excellence. This comprehensive cookbook is not just a collection of recipes; it is a fusion of science, nutrition, and culinary art designed to cater to the specific needs of individuals aiming to prevent or manage osteoporosis.

The foundation of this cookbook is built on the understanding that certain nutrients are crucial for bone health, including calcium, vitamin D, magnesium, potassium, and proteins. These nutrients play a vital role in maintaining bone density and strength, thereby reducing the risk of osteoporosis and fractures. The "Osteoporosis Diet Cookbook" offers a plethora of recipes rich in these essential nutrients, creatively incorporating them into delicious and easy-to-prepare meals suitable for daily consumption.

Each recipe in the cookbook is designed with simplicity and nutritional balance in mind, ensuring that users can enjoy a variety of flavors and cuisines while nurturing their bone health. From hearty breakfasts and nutrient-packed salads to satisfying main dishes and bone-friendly snacks, the "Osteoporosis Diet Cookbook" caters to all tastes and dietary preferences, including vegetarian, vegan, and gluten-free options.

The "Osteoporosis Diet Cookbook" is an invaluable resource for anyone seeking to enhance their bone health through diet. It combines nutritional guidance and culinary creativity to empower readers to make informed dietary choices that support strong, healthy bones. Whether you are looking to prevent osteoporosis or manage it, this cookbook is your companion on the journey to better bone health.

HAPPY COOKING!!!!!!

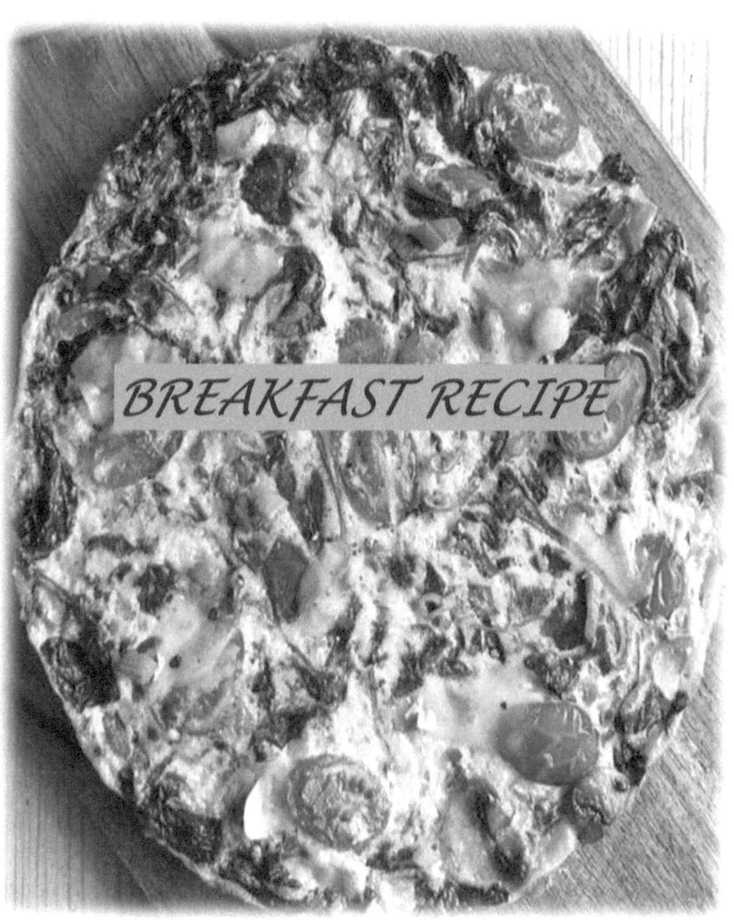
BREAKFAST RECIPE

RECIPES

BREAKFAST RECIPE

Spinach and Feta Omelet

Ingredients:

2 eggs

1 cup of fresh spinach

¼ cup of feta cheese

1 tbsp olive oil, salt, and

pepper.

Instructions:

In a pan, cook the spinach in olive oil until wilted.

Beat eggs and pour them over the spinach.

Add crumbled feta cheese on top.

Cook until the eggs are set, fold in half, and serve warm.

Savory Muffin Tin Quiches

Ingredients:

4 eggs

1 cup of chopped vegetables (e.g., bell peppers, onions, spinach)

½ cup of shredded cheese, and

¼ cup of milk.

Instructions:

Whisk together egg, milk, salt, and pepper.

Stir in vegetables and cheese.

Pour into greased muffin tins and bake at 375°F (190°C) for 20-25 minutes, or until set.

Salmon and Avocado Toast

Ingredients:

2 slices of whole-grain bread

1 ripe avocado

4 oz smoked salmon

1 tablespoon of lemon juice, and

Fresh dill.

Instructions:

Toast bread slices.

Mash avocado with lemon juice and spread on toast.

Top with smoked salmon and garnish with dill.

Salmon is high in vitamin D and omega-3 fatty acids.

Greek Yogurt Parfait

Ingredients:

1 cup of Greek yogurt (rich in protein and calcium)

½ cup of mixed berries (antioxidants)

¼ cup of granola (for crunch) and

A drizzle of honey.

Instructions:

Layer Greek yogurt, mixed berries, and granola in a glass.

Repeat the layers and top with a drizzle of honey for a sweet finish.

Almond Butter Banana Smoothie

Ingredients:

1 banana

2 tablespoons of almond butter

1 cup of fortified almond milk (high in calcium and vitamin D) and

A handful of spinach.

Instructions:

Blend all ingredients until smooth.

For a protein boost, add a scoop of your favorite protein powder.

Chia Seed Pudding

Ingredients:

¼ cup of chia seeds

1 cup of fortified plant-based milk

1 tablespoon of maple syrup, and

½ teaspoon of vanilla extract.

Instructions:

Mix all ingredients in a bowl.

Refrigerate overnight.

Serve topped with fresh fruit and a sprinkle of nuts for added calcium and healthy fats.

Sardine and Avocado Toast

Ingredients:

2 slices of whole-grain bread

1 ripe avocado

1 can of sardines in olive oil

lemon juice, and fresh parsley.

Instructions:

Mash avocado with lemon juice and spread on toasted bread.

Top with sardines and garnish with parsley.

Kale and Sweet Potato Hash

Ingredients:

1 large sweet potato (cubed)

2 cups of kale (chopped)

1 onion (chopped)

2 cloves of garlic (minced)

2 tablespoons of olive oil, salt, and pepper.

Instructions:

Sauté the onion and garlic in olive oil until transparent.

Add sweet potatoes and cook until tender.

Stir in kale and cook until wilted.

Season with salt and pepper.

Cottage Cheese and Peach Bowl

Ingredients:

1 cup of cottage cheese (high in calcium and protein)

1 sliced peach

A sprinkle of cinnamon, and

A handful of walnuts (for omega-3s).

Instructions:

Combine cottage cheese with sliced peach in a bowl.

Sprinkle with cinnamon and top with walnuts for a crunch.

Broccoli and Cheddar Cheese Oatmeal

Ingredients:

½ cup of rolled oats

1 cup of water or milk for cooking

1 cup of finely chopped broccoli (high in calcium)

¼ cup of shredded cheddar cheese (rich in calcium)

Salt, and pepper to taste.

Instructions:

Cook the oats in water or milk as per package instructions.

A few minutes before the oats are fully cooked, stir in the finely chopped broccoli.

Once cooked, mix in the shredded cheddar cheese until melted and season with salt and pepper.

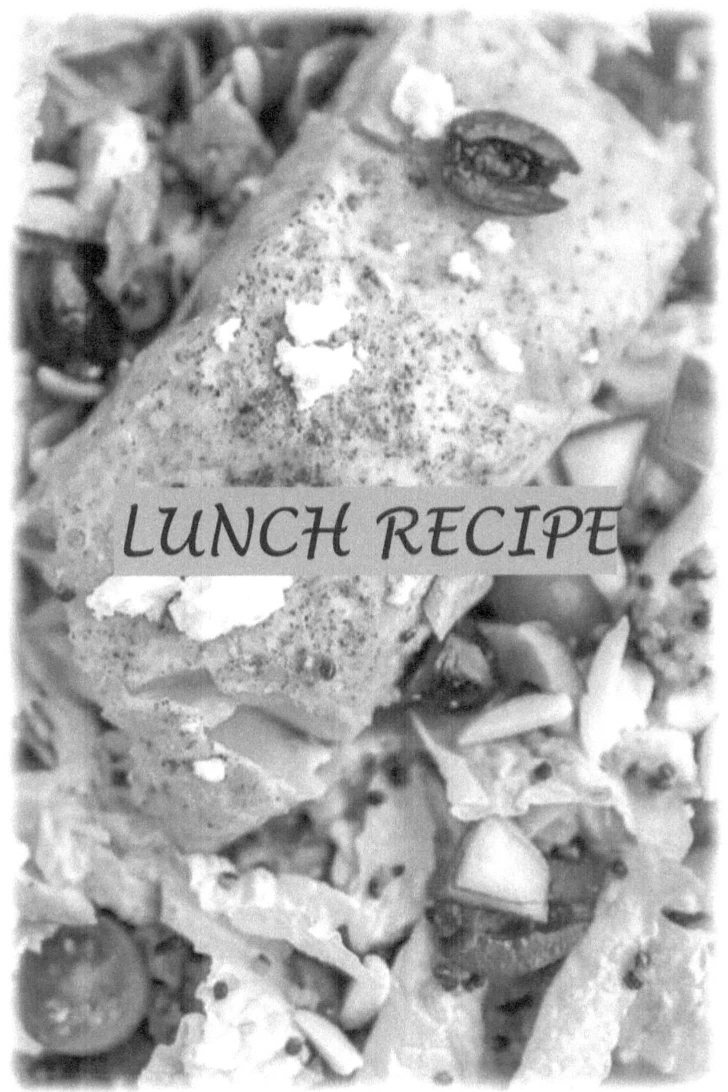
LUNCH RECIPE

LUNCH RECIPE

Grilled Salmon Salad

Ingredients:

4 oz salmon fillet

Mixed greens (spinach, arugula, kale)

Cherry tomatoes

Cucumber, and

A vinaigrette dressing.

Instructions:

Grill the salmon until fully cooked.

Combine the mixed greens, cherry tomatoes, and cucumber in a bowl.

Top with grilled salmon and drizzle with vinaigrette.

Chicken and Broccoli Stir-Fry

Ingredients:

1 chicken breast (cubed)

2 cups of broccoli florets

1 bell pepper (sliced)

2 tablespoons of soy sauce

1 tablespoon of sesame oil, and

1 clove of garlic (minced).

Instructions:

In a pan, heat sesame oil and sauté garlic until fragrant.

Add chicken and cook until browned.

Add broccoli and bell pepper, stir-frying until vegetables are tender.

Stir in soy sauce and cook for another minute.

Tofu and Kale Caesar Wrap

Ingredients:

1 cup of firm tofu (cubed and baked)

2 cups of kale (chopped)

whole grain wraps

Caesar dressing, and

Parmesan cheese.

Instructions:

Toss baked tofu and kale in Caesar dressing.

Lay the mixture on a whole grain wrap, sprinkle with

Parmesan cheese, and roll it up.

Lentil and Vegetable Soup

Ingredients:

1 cup of lentils

4 cups of vegetable broth

1 cup of diced tomatoes

2 carrots (chopped)

2 celery stalks (chopped)

1 onion (chopped), and

Spices (turmeric, cumin, salt, and pepper).

Instructions:

In a pot, combine all ingredients and bring to a boil.

Reduce heat and simmer until lentils and vegetables are tender.

Baked Cod with Almond Crust

Ingredients:

4 oz cod fillet

¼ cup of ground almonds

1 egg (beaten)

lemon zest, and

Parsley.

Instructions:

Dip the cod fillet in beaten egg

Then coat with ground almonds mixed with lemon zest and

parsley.

Bake at 400°F (200°C) for 10-12 minutes.

Spinach and Ricotta Stuffed Peppers

Ingredients:

2 bell peppers (halved and seeded)

1 cup of ricotta cheese

2 cups of spinach (chopped)

1 clove of garlic (minced), and

¼ cup of grated Parmesan cheese.

Instructions:

Mix ricotta, spinach, garlic, and half of the Parmesan.

Stuff the pepper halves with the mixture

Sprinkle the rest of the Parmesan on top

Bake at 375°F (190°C) for 25 minutes.

Turkey and Spinach Meatballs with Tomato Sauce

Ingredients:

1 lb. ground turkey

2 cups of spinach (finely chopped)

1 egg

2 tablespoons of whole grain breadcrumbs, and

1 jar of low-sodium tomato sauce.

Instructions:

Combine turkey, spinach, egg, and breadcrumbs.

Form into meatballs and bake at 375°F (190°C) for 20 minutes.

Heat tomato sauce and serve with meatballs.

Eggplant and Chickpea Stew

Ingredients:

1 eggplant (cubed)

1 can of chickpeas (drained)

1 can of diced tomatoes

1 onion (chopped)

2 cloves of garlic (minced), and

Spices (cumin, paprika, salt, and pepper).

Instructions:

Sauté onion and garlic until soft.

Add eggplant and cook until slightly tender.

Add chickpeas, tomatoes, and spices.

Simmer until flavors meld together.

Roasted Beet and Goat Cheese Salad

Ingredients:

2 beets (roasted and sliced)

mixed greens

½ cup of goat cheese (crumbled)

¼ cup of walnuts (toasted), and

Balsamic vinaigrette.

Instructions:

Toss mixed greens with balsamic vinaigrette.

Top with sliced beets, crumbled goat cheese, and toasted walnuts.

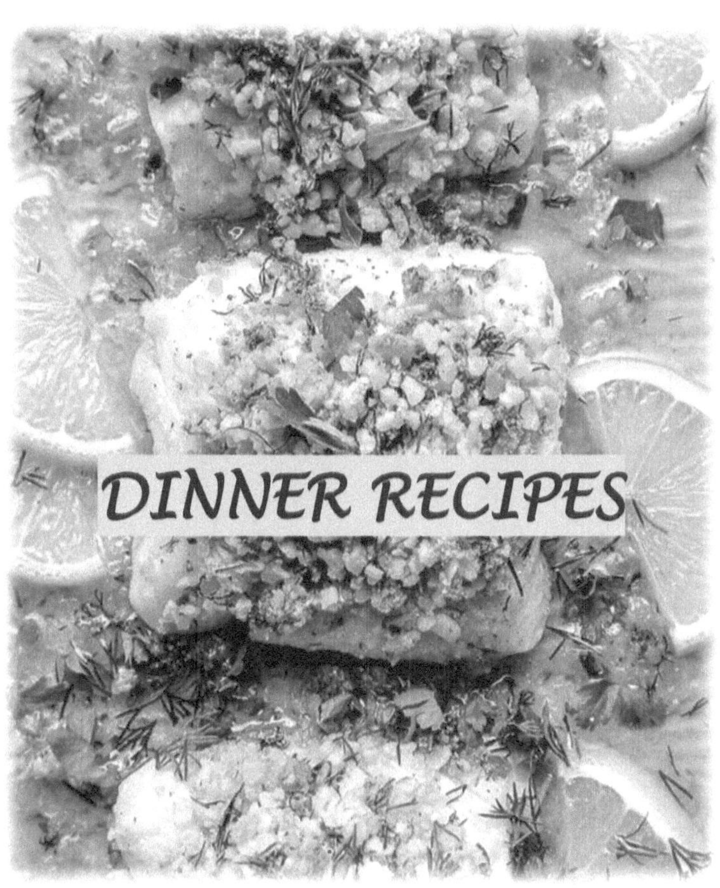

DINNER RECIPES

DINNER RECIPE

Baked Salmon with Lemon and Dill

Ingredients:

2 salmon fillets

1 lemon (sliced)

Fresh dill

Olive oil

Salt, and

pepper.

Instructions:

Place salmon on a baking sheet, season with salt and pepper,

Top with lemon slices and dill.

Drizzle with olive oil

Bake at 400°F (200°C) for 12-15 minutes.

Stuffed Chicken Breast with Spinach and Feta

Ingredients:

2 chicken breasts

1 cup of spinach

½ cup of feta cheese

1 clove of garlic (minced)

Salt, and

Pepper.

Instructions:

Make a pocket in each chicken breast.

Mix spinach, feta, and garlic, then stuff into chicken.

Season with salt and pepper

Bake at 375°F (190°C) for 25 minutes.

Roasted Vegetable and Chickpea Bowl

Ingredients:

1 sweet potato (cubed)

1 bell pepper (sliced)

1 zucchini (sliced)

1 cup of chickpeas (drained)

Olive oil

Cumin

Paprika

Salt, and

Pepper.

Instructions:

Toss vegetables and chickpeas with olive oil, cumin, paprika, salt, and pepper.

Roast at 425°F (220°C) for 25-30 minutes.

Turkey Chili with Beans

Ingredients:

1 lb. ground turkey

1 can of kidney beans (drained)

1 can of diced tomatoes

1 onion (chopped)

1 bell pepper (chopped)

Chili powder

Cumin, and

Garlic powder.

Instructions:

Brown turkey with onion and bell pepper.

Add beans, tomatoes, and spices.

Simmer for 30 minutes.

Eggplant Parmesan

Ingredients:

1 eggplant (sliced and salted)

2 cups of marinara sauce

1 cup of shredded mozzarella

½ cup of grated Parmesan, breadcrumbs, and

Olive oil.

Instructions:

Rinse eggplant slices and coat with breadcrumbs.

Fry until golden.

In a baking dish, layer eggplant, marinara, and cheeses.

Bake at 375°F (190°C) for 30 minutes.

Grilled Shrimp and Asparagus

Ingredients:

1 lb. shrimp (peeled and deveined)

2 cups of asparagus (trimmed)

olive oil

lemon juice

garlic (minced)

Salt, and pepper.

Instructions:

Marinate shrimp and asparagus in olive oil, lemon juice, garlic, salt, and pepper.

Grill until shrimp is pink and asparagus is tender.

Broccoli and Cauliflower Gratin

Ingredients:

2 cups of broccoli (chopped)

2 cups of cauliflower (chopped)

1 cup of heavy cream

½ cup of grated cheese (choose a high-calcium variety)

Breadcrumbs

Salt, and pepper.

Instructions:

Blanch broccoli and cauliflower.

Layer in a baking dish, pour over cream, sprinkle with cheese and breadcrumbs.

Bake at 375°F (190°C) until golden.

Beef and Broccoli Stir-Fry

Ingredients:

1 lb. beef strips

2 cups of broccoli florets

1 onion (sliced)

2 cloves of garlic (minced)

Soy sauce

Sesame oil, and

Cornstarch.

Instructions:

Marinate beef in soy sauce sesame oil, and cornstarch.

Stir-fry beef until browned, set aside.

Stir-fry broccoli and onion, add garlic

Reintroduce beef and heat through.

Ricotta and Spinach Stuffed Portobello Mushrooms

Ingredients:

4 large Portobello mushrooms

1 cup of ricotta cheese

1 cup of spinach (chopped)

¼ cup of grated Parmesan

1 clove of garlic (minced)

Salt, and pepper.

Instructions:

Remove mushroom stems and scrape gills.

Mix ricotta, spinach, Parmesan, garlic, salt, and pepper.

Stuff mushrooms, bake at 375°F (190°C) for 20 minutes.

Lemon Garlic Tilapia

Ingredients:

4 tilapia fillets

2 lemons (1 sliced, 1 juiced)

2 cloves of garlic (minced)

Parsley (chopped)

Olive oil

Salt, and pepper.

Instructions:

Place tilapia on a baking sheet.

Season with salt, pepper, lemon juice, and garlic.

Top with lemon slices and parsley.

Drizzle with olive oil.

Bake at 400°F (200°C) for 10-12 minutes.

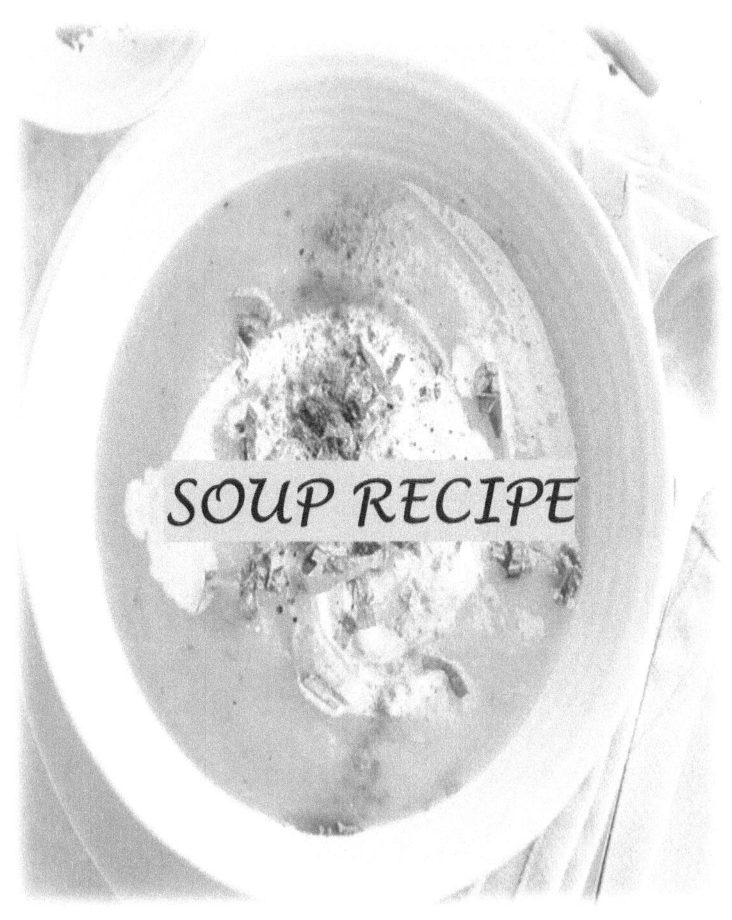
SOUP RECIPE

SOUP RECIPE

Creamy Broccoli and Spinach Soup

Ingredients:

2 cups broccoli florets

1 cup fresh spinach

1 onion (chopped)

2 cloves garlic (minced)

4 cups vegetable broth

1 cup heavy cream

Salt, and pepper to taste.

Instructions:

Sauté onion and garlic until translucent.

Add broccoli and vegetable broth, simmering until broccoli is tender.

Add spinach, cooking until wilted.

Blend until smooth, return to heat, and stir in heavy cream.

Season with salt and pepper.

Roasted Butternut Squash Soup

Ingredients:

1 butternut squash (peeled and cubed)

1 onion (chopped)

3 cups vegetable broth

1 tsp cinnamon

½ cup coconut milk

 Salt, and pepper to taste.

Instructions:

Roast butternut squash at 400°F (200°C) until tender.

Sauté onion, add roasted squash, vegetable broth, and cinnamon.

Simmer for 20 minutes, blend until smooth, and stir in coconut milk.

Season with salt and pepper.

Chicken and Kale Soup

Ingredients:

1 lb. chicken breast (cubed)

2 cups kale (chopped)

1 onion (chopped),

2 carrots (chopped)

2 celery stalks (chopped)

4 cups chicken broth

Salt, and pepper to taste.

Instructions:

Sauté onion, carrots, and celery.

Add chicken and broth, simmer until chicken is cooked.

Add kale in the last 5 minutes.

Season with salt and pepper.

Lentil and Tomato Soup

Ingredients:

1 cup lentils

1 can diced tomatoes

1 onion (chopped)

2 carrots (chopped)

4 cups vegetable broth

1 tsp turmeric

Salt, and pepper to taste.

Instructions:

Sauté onion and carrots until tender.

Add lentils, tomatoes, broth, and turmeric.

Simmer until lentils are soft.

Season with salt and pepper.

Miso Soup with Tofu and Seaweed

Ingredients:

4 cups water

3 tbsp miso paste

½ block firm tofu (cubed)

1 cup seaweed (chopped)

2 green onions (chopped).

Instructions:

Dissolve miso paste in water over low heat.

Add tofu and seaweed, simmering for 5 minutes.

Garnish with green onions before serving.

White Bean and Escarole Soup

Ingredients:

1 can white beans (drained and rinsed)

1 head escarole (chopped)

1 onion (chopped)

4 cups vegetable broth

1 parmesan rind (optional)

Salt, and pepper to taste.

Instructions:

Sauté onion until translucent.

Add beans, escarole, broth, and parmesan rind.

Simmer until escarole is wilted.

Remove parmesan rind, season with salt and pepper.

Carrot Ginger Soup

Ingredients:

2 lbs. carrots (peeled and chopped)

1 onion (chopped)

2 tbsp ginger (minced)

4 cups vegetable broth

1 cup orange juice

Salt, and pepper to taste.

Instructions:

Sauté onion and ginger until fragrant.

Add carrots and broth, simmering until carrots are tender.

Blend until smooth, stir in orange juice, and season with salt
and pepper.

Beet and Cabbage Borscht

Ingredients:

3 beets (peeled and grated)

½ head cabbage (shredded)

1 onion (chopped)

4 cups vegetable broth

2 tbsp apple cider vinegar

Salt, and pepper to taste.

Instructions:

Sauté onion, add beets, cabbage, and broth.

Simmer until vegetables are tender.

Stir in vinegar, season with salt and pepper.

Pumpkin Coconut Soup

Ingredients:

2 cups pumpkin puree

1 onion (chopped)

4 cups vegetable broth

1 tsp curry powder

½ cup coconut milk

Salt, and pepper to taste.

Instructions:

Sauté onion, add pumpkin puree, broth, and curry powder.

Simmer for 20 minutes.

Blend until smooth, stir in coconut milk

Season with salt and pepper.

Spinach and White Bean Soup

Ingredients:

2 cups spinach (chopped)

1 can white beans (drained and rinsed)

1 onion (chopped)

3 cloves garlic (minced)

4 cups vegetable broth

1 lemon (juice and zest)

Salt, and pepper to taste.

Instructions:

Sauté onion and garlic until translucent.

Add beans, broth, and lemon zest.

Simmer for 10 minutes.

Add spinach and cook until wilted.

Stir in lemon juice, season with salt and pepper.

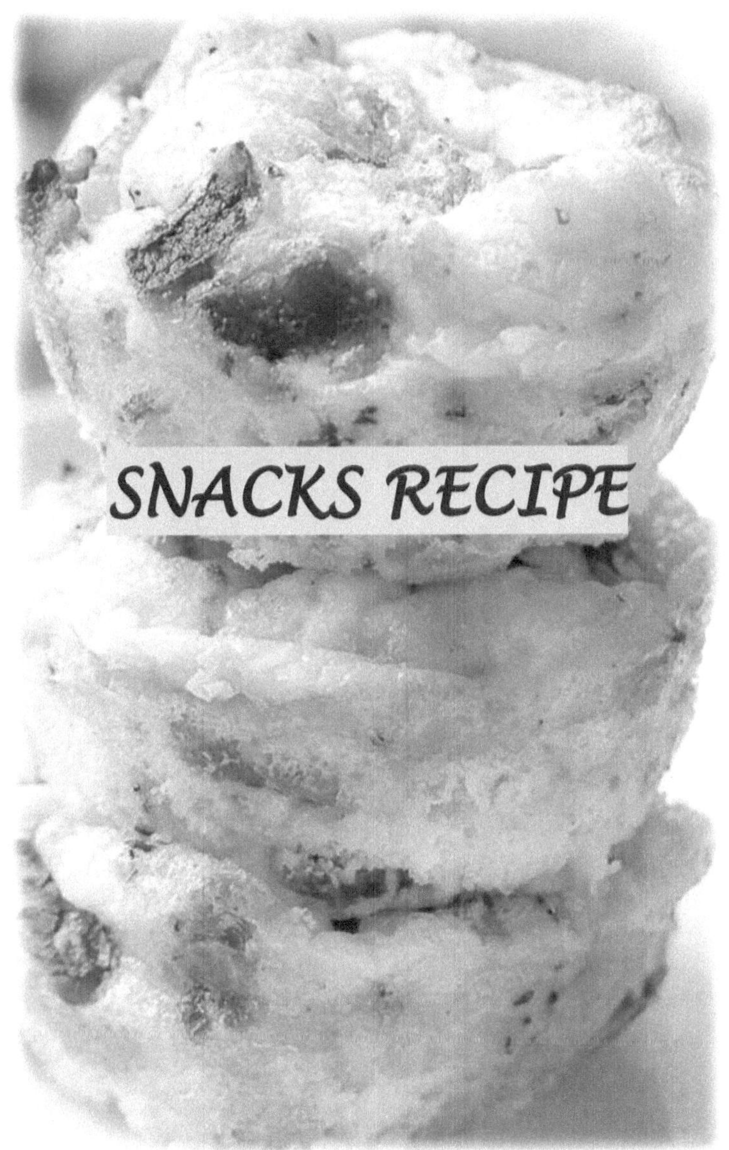

SNACKS RECIPE

SNACKS RECIPE

Greek Yogurt with Almonds and Honey

Ingredients:

1 cup plain Greek yogurt

A handful of almonds

1 tablespoon honey

Instructions:

Spoon Greek yogurt into a bowl.

Top with almonds and drizzle with honey.

Chia Seed Pudding

Ingredients:

2 tablespoons chia seeds

½ cup almond milk

1 tablespoon maple syrup

½ cup fresh berries.

Instructions:

Mix chia seeds, almond milk, and maple syrup in a bowl.

Refrigerate overnight.

Top with fresh berries before serving.

Kale Chips

Ingredients:

1 bunch kale

1 tablespoon olive oil

Sea salt to taste.

Instructions:

Preheat oven to 350°F (175°C).

Remove the kale stems and shred the leaves into bite-sized
pieces.

Toss with olive oil and salt.

Spread on a baking sheet and bake for 10-15 minutes until
crispy.

Cheese and Apple Slices

Ingredients:

1 apple

1 ounce cheese (such as cheddar or gouda).

Instructions:

Slice the apple.

Cut cheese into thin slices.

Pair each apple slice with a slice of cheese.

Roasted Edamame

Ingredients:

1 cup shelled edamame

Olive oil spray

Sea salt to taste.

Instructions:

Preheat oven to 375°F (190°C).

Spray edamame lightly with olive oil and sprinkle with sea salt.

Roast for 10-15 minutes until crispy.

Cottage Cheese with Pineapple

Ingredients:

½ cup cottage cheese

½ cup chopped pineapple.

Instructions:

Combine cottage cheese and pineapple in a bowl.

Mix gently.

Carrot Sticks with Hummus

Ingredients:

2 large carrots

¼ cup hummus.

Instructions:

Cut carrots into sticks.

Serve with hummus for dipping.

Tuna Salad on Cucumber Slices

Ingredients:

1 can tuna (drained)

1 tablespoon yogurt

1 cucumber.

Instructions:

Mix tuna with yogurt.

Slice cucumber into rounds.

Top each cucumber slice with a spoonful of tuna salad.

Hard-Boiled Eggs

Ingredients:

2 eggs.

Instructions:

Place eggs in a saucepan and cover with water.

Bring to a boil, then cover and turn off the heat.

Let sit for 12 minutes.

Cool in cold water, peel, and serve.

Ricotta and Fig Spread on Whole Grain Crackers

Ingredients:

½ cup ricotta cheese

2 tablespoons fig spread

Whole grain crackers.

Instructions:

Spread ricotta cheese on crackers.

Top each with a small dollop of fig spread.

CONCLUSION

We have ventured beyond mere dietary guidelines, turning the spotlight on how food can be both medicine and joy. The importance of incorporating a variety of foods, each playing a unique role in bone health, has been a recurring theme. Through creative use of ingredients like leafy greens, dairy products, nuts, seeds, and lean proteins, we've laid out a path that doesn't just aim to prevent or manage osteoporosis but also enhances overall well-being.

The journey doesn't end with the last recipe in this book. It's a continuous exploration of how dietary choices can influence our health. We encourage readers to experiment with the recipes, tweak them to personal tastes and nutritional needs, and make them a part of a balanced lifestyle that includes regular physical activity and exposure to sunlight for natural vitamin D.

Remember, the fight against osteoporosis is multifaceted, involving more than just diet. Consistent exercise, regular check-ups with healthcare providers, and a holistic approach to wellness are pivotal.

This cookbook is a tool—one of many in your arsenal—to help fortify your bones and enhance your life quality.

As you close this book, let the journey of nurturing your bones through mindful eating continue. Let each meal be a step toward stronger bones, a healthier body, and a happier you. Here's to your health, your vitality, and a future where osteoporosis is not a limitation but a challenge met with knowledge, flavor, and joy.

DAILY MEAL PLANNER

DAILY —

Meal Planner

Date: ....

Breakfast

Grocery List

☐ ______________________

☐ ______________________

☐ ______________________

☐ ______________________

☐ ______________________

☐ ______________________

☐ ______________________

☐ ______________________

☐ ______________________

Lunch

Dinner

Notes

Snack

DAILY —
Meal Planner
Date:

Breakfast

Grocery List

Lunch

Dinner

Notes

Snack

Meal Planner

Date: ....

Breakfast

Lunch

Dinner

Snack

Grocery List

Notes

DAILY —

Meal Planner

Date: ....

Breakfast	Grocery List

☐
☐
☐
☐
☐
☐
☐
☐
☐

Lunch

Dinner

Notes

Snack

Meal Planner

Date: ....

Breakfast

Lunch

Dinner

Snack

Grocery List

- ☐
- ☐
- ☐
- ☐
- ☐
- ☐
- ☐
- ☐
- ☐

Notes

Meal Planner

DAILY —

Date: ....

Breakfast

Lunch

Dinner

Snack

Grocery List

☐
☐
☐
☐
☐
☐
☐
☐
☐

Notes

DAILY —

Meal Planner

Date:

Breakfast

Lunch

Dinner

Snack

Grocery List

☐
☐
☐
☐
☐
☐
☐
☐
☐

Notes

Meal Planner

Date: ....

Breakfast

Grocery List

☐
☐
☐
☐
☐
☐
☐
☐
☐

Lunch

Dinner

Notes

Snack

Meal Planner

Date: ....

Breakfast

Lunch

Dinner

Snack

Grocery List

Notes

Meal Planner

Date:

Breakfast

Grocery List

☐
☐
☐
☐
☐
☐
☐
☐
☐

Lunch

Dinner

Notes

Snack

Meal Planner

Date: ....

Breakfast

Lunch

Dinner

Snack

Grocery List

- [ ]
- [ ]
- [ ]
- [ ]
- [ ]
- [ ]
- [ ]
- [ ]
- [ ]

Notes

DAILY —

Meal Planner

Date: ....

Breakfast

Lunch

Dinner

Snack

Grocery List

- ☐
- ☐
- ☐
- ☐
- ☐
- ☐
- ☐
- ☐
- ☐

Notes

Meal Planner

Date: ....

Breakfast

Grocery List

☐
☐
☐
☐
☐
☐
☐
☐
☐

Lunch

Dinner

Snack

Notes

DAILY —

Meal Planner

Date:

Breakfast

Lunch

Dinner

Snack

Grocery List

Notes

DAILY —
Meal Planner
Date:
Breakfast
Lunch
Dinner
Snack
Grocery List
Notes

Meal Planner

Date: ....

Breakfast	Grocery List

Lunch

Dinner

Snack

Notes

DAILY —

Meal Planner

Date:

Breakfast

Lunch

Dinner

Snack

Grocery List

Notes

Meal Planner

Date: ....

Breakfast

Grocery List

Lunch

Dinner

Notes

Snack

DAILY —

Meal Planner

Date: ....

Breakfast

Lunch

Dinner

Snack

Grocery List

☐
☐
☐
☐
☐
☐
☐
☐
☐

Notes

Meal Planner

Date: ....

Breakfast

Lunch

Dinner

Snack

Grocery List

Notes

DAILY —

Meal Planner

Date: ....

Breakfast

Grocery List

☐
☐
☐
☐
☐
☐
☐
☐
☐

Lunch

Dinner

Notes

Snack

Meal Planner

Date: ....

Breakfast

Grocery List

☐ ____________
☐ ____________
☐ ____________
☐ ____________
☐ ____________
☐ ____________
☐ ____________
☐ ____________
☐ ____________

Lunch

Dinner

Notes

Snack

Meal Planner

Date: ....

Breakfast

Lunch

Dinner

Snack

Grocery List

- [ ]
- [ ]
- [ ]
- [ ]
- [ ]
- [ ]
- [ ]
- [ ]
- [ ]

Notes

DAILY —
Meal Planner

Date:

Breakfast

Grocery List

Lunch

Dinner

Notes

Snack

Meal Planner

Date: ....

Breakfast

____

____

____

Lunch

____

____

____

Dinner

____

____

____

Snack

____

____

____

Grocery List

☐ ____________________

☐ ____________________

☐ ____________________

☐ ____________________

☐ ____________________

☐ ____________________

☐ ____________________

☐ ____________________

☐ ____________________

Notes

____

____

____

____

____

____

____

DAILY —
Meal Planner
Date:
Breakfast
Grocery List
Lunch
Dinner
Snack
Notes

Meal Planner

Date: ....

Breakfast	Grocery List
	☐
	☐

Lunch

Dinner

Snack

Notes

Meal Planner

Date: ....

Breakfast

Lunch

Dinner

Snack

Grocery List

- ☐
- ☐
- ☐
- ☐
- ☐
- ☐
- ☐
- ☐
- ☐

Notes

DAILY —

Meal Planner

Date: ....

Breakfast

Grocery List
☐ ________________________
☐ ________________________
☐ ________________________
☐ ________________________
☐ ________________________
☐ ________________________
☐ ________________________
☐ ________________________
☐ ________________________

Lunch

Dinner

Notes

Snack

www.ingramcontent.com/pod-product-compliance
Lightning Source LLC
Chambersburg PA
CBHW031319250726
48656CB00005B/1877